Week Starting:

	AM Blood Sugar Reading	PM Blood Sugar Reading	Gastroparesis Symptoms	Foods preceding symptoms
Sunday				
Monday				
Tuesday				
Wednesday				
Thursday				
Friday				
Saturday				

	Week Starting:			

	AM Blood Sugar Reading	**PM Blood Sugar Reading**	**Gastroparesis Symptoms**	**Foods preceding symptoms**
Sunday				
Monday				
Tuesday				
Wednesday				
Thursday				
Friday				
Saturday				

	AM Blood Sugar Reading	PM Blood Sugar Reading	Gastroparesis Symptoms	Foods preceding symptoms
Week Starting:				
Sunday				
Monday				
Tuesday				
Wednesday				
Thursday				
Friday				
Saturday				

	AM Blood Sugar Reading	PM Blood Sugar Reading	Gastroparesis Symptoms	Foods preceding symptoms
Sunday				
Monday				
Tuesday				
Wednesday				
Thursday				
Friday				
Saturday				

Week Starting:				
	AM Blood Sugar Reading	PM Blood Sugar Reading	Gastroparesis Symptoms	Foods preceding symptoms
Sunday				
Monday				
Tuesday				
Wednesday				
Thursday				
Friday				
Saturday				

	AM Blood Sugar Reading	PM Blood Sugar Reading	Gastroparesis Symptoms	Foods preceding symptoms
Week Starting:				
Sunday				
Monday				
Tuesday				
Wednesday				
Thursday				
Friday				
Saturday				

	AM Blood Sugar Reading	PM Blood Sugar Reading	Gastroparesis Symptoms	Foods preceding symptoms
Sunday				
Monday				
Tuesday				
Wednesday				
Thursday				
Friday				
Saturday				

Week Starting:				
	AM Blood Sugar Reading	PM Blood Sugar Reading	Gastroparesis Symptoms	Foods preceding symptoms
Sunday				
Monday				
Tuesday				
Wednesday				
Thursday				
Friday				
Saturday				

Week Starting:				
	AM Blood Sugar Reading	PM Blood Sugar Reading	Gastroparesis Symptoms	Foods preceding symptoms
Sunday				
Monday				
Tuesday				
Wednesday				
Thursday				
Friday				
Saturday				

Week Starting:				
	AM Blood Sugar Reading	PM Blood Sugar Reading	Gastroparesis Symptoms	Foods preceding symptoms
Sunday				
Monday				
Tuesday				
Wednesday				
Thursday				
Friday				
Saturday				

Week Starting:				

	AM Blood Sugar Reading	PM Blood Sugar Reading	Gastroparesis Symptoms	Foods preceding symptoms
Sunday				
Monday				
Tuesday				
Wednesday				
Thursday				
Friday				
Saturday				

	AM Blood Sugar Reading	PM Blood Sugar Reading	Gastroparesis Symptoms	Foods preceding symptoms
Sunday				
Monday				
Tuesday				
Wednesday				
Thursday				
Friday				
Saturday				

Week Starting:				
	AM Blood Sugar Reading	PM Blood Sugar Reading	Gastroparesis Symptoms	Foods preceding symptoms
Sunday				
Monday				
Tuesday				
Wednesday				
Thursday				
Friday				
Saturday				

	AM Blood Sugar Reading	PM Blood Sugar Reading	Gastroparesis Symptoms	Foods preceding symptoms
Week Starting:				
Sunday				
Monday				
Tuesday				
Wednesday				
Thursday				
Friday				
Saturday				

Week Starting:

	AM Blood Sugar Reading	PM Blood Sugar Reading	Gastroparesis Symptoms	Foods preceding symptoms
Sunday				
Monday				
Tuesday				
Wednesday				
Thursday				
Friday				
Saturday				

	Week Starting:			

	AM Blood Sugar Reading	PM Blood Sugar Reading	Gastroparesis Symptoms	Foods preceding symptoms
Sunday				
Monday				
Tuesday				
Wednesday				
Thursday				
Friday				
Saturday				

	AM Blood Sugar Reading	PM Blood Sugar Reading	Gastroparesis Symptoms	Foods preceding symptoms
Week Starting:				
Sunday				
Monday				
Tuesday				
Wednesday				
Thursday				
Friday				
Saturday				

	AM Blood Sugar Reading	**PM Blood Sugar Reading**	**Gastroparesis Symptoms**	**Foods preceding symptoms**
Sunday				
Monday				
Tuesday				
Wednesday				
Thursday				
Friday				
Saturday				

Week Starting:

Week Starting:

	AM Blood Sugar Reading	PM Blood Sugar Reading	Gastroparesis Symptoms	Foods preceding symptoms
Sunday				
Monday				
Tuesday				
Wednesday				
Thursday				
Friday				
Saturday				

Week Starting:

	AM Blood Sugar Reading	PM Blood Sugar Reading	Gastroparesis Symptoms	Foods preceding symptoms
Sunday				
Monday				
Tuesday				
Wednesday				
Thursday				
Friday				
Saturday				

Week Starting:

	AM Blood Sugar Reading	PM Blood Sugar Reading	Gastroparesis Symptoms	Foods preceding symptoms
Sunday				
Monday				
Tuesday				
Wednesday				
Thursday				
Friday				
Saturday				

	AM Blood Sugar Reading	PM Blood Sugar Reading	Gastroparesis Symptoms	Foods preceding symptoms
Sunday				
Monday				
Tuesday				
Wednesday				
Thursday				
Friday				
Saturday				

	AM Blood Sugar Reading	PM Blood Sugar Reading	Gastroparesis Symptoms	Foods preceding symptoms
Sunday				
Monday				
Tuesday				
Wednesday				
Thursday				
Friday				
Saturday				

Week Starting:

	AM Blood Sugar Reading	PM Blood Sugar Reading	Gastroparesis Symptoms	Foods preceding symptoms
Sunday				
Monday				
Tuesday				
Wednesday				
Thursday				
Friday				
Saturday				

Week Starting:				

	AM Blood Sugar Reading	PM Blood Sugar Reading	Gastroparesis Symptoms	Foods preceding symptoms
Sunday				
Monday				
Tuesday				
Wednesday				
Thursday				
Friday				
Saturday				

Week Starting:				
	AM Blood Sugar Reading	PM Blood Sugar Reading	Gastroparesis Symptoms	Foods preceding symptoms
Sunday				
Monday				
Tuesday				
Wednesday				
Thursday				
Friday				
Saturday				

| Week Starting: |

	AM Blood Sugar Reading	PM Blood Sugar Reading	Gastroparesis Symptoms	Foods preceding symptoms
Sunday				
Monday				
Tuesday				
Wednesday				
Thursday				
Friday				
Saturday				

	AM Blood Sugar Reading	PM Blood Sugar Reading	Gastroparesis Symptoms	Foods preceding symptoms
Sunday				
Monday				
Tuesday				
Wednesday				
Thursday				
Friday				
Saturday				

Week Starting:				

	AM Blood Sugar Reading	PM Blood Sugar Reading	Gastroparesis Symptoms	Foods preceding symptoms
Sunday				
Monday				
Tuesday				
Wednesday				
Thursday				
Friday				
Saturday				

Week Starting:				

	AM Blood Sugar Reading	PM Blood Sugar Reading	Gastroparesis Symptoms	Foods preceding symptoms
Sunday				
Monday				
Tuesday				
Wednesday				
Thursday				
Friday				
Saturday				

Week Starting:				
	AM Blood Sugar Reading	PM Blood Sugar Reading	Gastroparesis Symptoms	Foods preceding symptoms
Sunday				
Monday				
Tuesday				
Wednesday				
Thursday				
Friday				
Saturday				

	AM Blood Sugar Reading	PM Blood Sugar Reading	Gastroparesis Symptoms	Foods preceding symptoms
Sunday				
Monday				
Tuesday				
Wednesday				
Thursday				
Friday				
Saturday				

Week Starting:

Week Starting:				

	AM Blood Sugar Reading	PM Blood Sugar Reading	Gastroparesis Symptoms	Foods preceding symptoms
Sunday				
Monday				
Tuesday				
Wednesday				
Thursday				
Friday				
Saturday				

Week Starting:				

	AM Blood Sugar Reading	PM Blood Sugar Reading	Gastroparesis Symptoms	Foods preceding symptoms
Sunday				
Monday				
Tuesday				
Wednesday				
Thursday				
Friday				
Saturday				

	AM Blood Sugar Reading	PM Blood Sugar Reading	Gastroparesis Symptoms	Foods preceding symptoms
Sunday				
Monday				
Tuesday				
Wednesday				
Thursday				
Friday				
Saturday				

	AM Blood Sugar Reading	PM Blood Sugar Reading	Gastroparesis Symptoms	Foods preceding symptoms
Sunday				
Monday				
Tuesday				
Wednesday				
Thursday				
Friday				
Saturday				

Week Starting:

Week Starting:				
	AM Blood Sugar Reading	PM Blood Sugar Reading	Gastroparesis Symptoms	Foods preceding symptoms
Sunday				
Monday				
Tuesday				
Wednesday				
Thursday				
Friday				
Saturday				

	AM Blood Sugar Reading	PM Blood Sugar Reading	Gastroparesis Symptoms	Foods preceding symptoms
Week Starting:				
Sunday				
Monday				
Tuesday				
Wednesday				
Thursday				
Friday				
Saturday				

	AM Blood Sugar Reading	PM Blood Sugar Reading	Gastroparesis Symptoms	Foods preceding symptoms
Sunday				
Monday				
Tuesday				
Wednesday				
Thursday				
Friday				
Saturday				

Week Starting:

Week Starting:

	AM Blood Sugar Reading	PM Blood Sugar Reading	Gastroparesis Symptoms	Foods preceding symptoms
Sunday				
Monday				
Tuesday				
Wednesday				
Thursday				
Friday				
Saturday				

Week Starting:

	AM Blood Sugar Reading	PM Blood Sugar Reading	Gastroparesis Symptoms	Foods preceding symptoms
Sunday				
Monday				
Tuesday				
Wednesday				
Thursday				
Friday				
Saturday				

Week Starting:				
	AM Blood Sugar Reading	**PM Blood Sugar Reading**	**Gastroparesis Symptoms**	**Foods preceding symptoms**
Sunday				
Monday				
Tuesday				
Wednesday				
Thursday				
Friday				
Saturday				

Week Starting:

	AM Blood Sugar Reading	PM Blood Sugar Reading	Gastroparesis Symptoms	Foods preceding symptoms
Sunday				
Monday				
Tuesday				
Wednesday				
Thursday				
Friday				
Saturday				

Week Starting:

	AM Blood Sugar Reading	PM Blood Sugar Reading	Gastroparesis Symptoms	Foods preceding symptoms
Sunday				
Monday				
Tuesday				
Wednesday				
Thursday				
Friday				
Saturday				

	AM Blood Sugar Reading	PM Blood Sugar Reading	Gastroparesis Symptoms	Foods preceding symptoms
Sunday				
Monday				
Tuesday				
Wednesday				
Thursday				
Friday				
Saturday				

Week Starting:				
	AM Blood Sugar Reading	PM Blood Sugar Reading	Gastroparesis Symptoms	Foods preceding symptoms
Sunday				
Monday				
Tuesday				
Wednesday				
Thursday				
Friday				
Saturday				

Week Starting:

	AM Blood Sugar Reading	PM Blood Sugar Reading	Gastroparesis Symptoms	Foods preceding symptoms
Sunday				
Monday				
Tuesday				
Wednesday				
Thursday				
Friday				
Saturday				

Week Starting:				
	AM Blood Sugar Reading	**PM Blood Sugar Reading**	**Gastroparesis Symptoms**	**Foods preceding symptoms**
Sunday				
Monday				
Tuesday				
Wednesday				
Thursday				
Friday				
Saturday				

Week Starting:				
	AM Blood Sugar Reading	PM Blood Sugar Reading	Gastroparesis Symptoms	Foods preceding symptoms
Sunday				
Monday				
Tuesday				
Wednesday				
Thursday				
Friday				
Saturday				

Week Starting:

	AM Blood Sugar Reading	PM Blood Sugar Reading	Gastroparesis Symptoms	Foods preceding symptoms
Sunday				
Monday				
Tuesday				
Wednesday				
Thursday				
Friday				
Saturday				

	AM Blood Sugar Reading	PM Blood Sugar Reading	Gastroparesis Symptoms	Foods preceding symptoms
Sunday				
Monday				
Tuesday				
Wednesday				
Thursday				
Friday				
Saturday				

Week Starting:

	Week Starting:			

	AM Blood Sugar Reading	**PM Blood Sugar Reading**	**Gastroparesis Symptoms**	**Foods preceding symptoms**
Sunday				
Monday				
Tuesday				
Wednesday				
Thursday				
Friday				
Saturday				

Made in the USA
Monee, IL
02 April 2023

31081971R00031